# Acceptance Groups
*for*
*Survivors*

## A Guide for Facilitators

*by Nancy Bauser M.S.W., A.C.S.W.*

*Based on the life experience of a brain-injury survivor, this structured group program is designed to help people with disabilities accept themselves and their new life circumstances*

**Intended for use by rehabilitation professionals who work with survivors of traumatic brain injuries or other conditions resulting in disabilities**

© 2000, 2001 by Nancy Bauser M.S.W., A.C.S.W.
All rights reserved.
No part of this book may be reproduced, stored in a retrieval system, or transmitted by any means, electronic, mechanical, photocopying, recording, or otherwise, without written permission from the author.

ISBN 0-75962-263-9

This book is printed on acid free paper.

Library of Congress number: TXu 951 – 830

1stBooks – rev. 9/5/01

This book is dedicated to my husband Bill, who gives me what I need when I need it and then urges me on.

A special thanks to Isabelle M. Davis for her editorial expertise and friendship.

# Table of Contents

*Table of Contents*......................................................*v*

*Introduction*............................................................*ix*

*Objectives of Acceptance Groups for Survivors*. *xi*

*A Message from the Author*..................................*xv*

*Guidelines for Facilitators*................................*xxiii*

*Part I — Dealing with Me*........................................ *1*

    Week 1:   Meanings of Acceptance and Recovery...................................................... 5

    Week 2:   Expectations of Self....................... 7

    Week 3:   Physical Limitations As a Result of Injury/Disability/Illness........................ 11

    Week 4:   Healthy Problem Solving............ 13

    Week 5:   Living with an Injury/Disability/Illness............................ 17

    Week 6:   Dealing with Me — Review Weeks 1 to 5............................................... 21

*Part II — Dealing With Others* .......................... *23*

    Week 7:    Getting Back to Work ................. 27

    Week 8:    Support Systems ......................... 29

    Week 9:    Asking for Assistance ................. 31

    Week 10:  Relating to Others ....................... 35

    Week 11:  Requiring Assistance ................... 39

    Week 12:  Dealing With Others — Review
                 Weeks 7 to 11 ............................................ 43

*Part III — Dealing with Feelings* ....................... *47*

    Week 13:  Feelings about Being
                 Injured/Disabled/Ill ............................... 51

    Week 14:  Feeling OK Today ....................... 53

    Week 15:  Feelings About Self ..................... 55

    Week 16:  Loss and Acceptance .................. 57

    Week 17:  Expressing Uncomfortable
                 Feelings ....................................................... 61

    Week 18:  Dealing With Feelings — Review
                 Weeks 13 to 17 ........................................ 65

*Part IV — Putting It Together*............................ *68*

   **Week 19: Feeling Good About Yourself.... 71**

   **Week 20: Possibilities After**

          **Injury/Disability/Illness ........................... 73**

   **Week 21: Disability and the Workplace.... 75**

   **Week 22: Setting Limits............................... 77**

   **Week 23: Accepting Yourself — Just the**

          **Way You Are .............................................. 79**

   **Week 24: Putting It Together — Review**

          **Weeks 19 to 23 ........................................... 83**

*About the Author .................................................. 89*

# Introduction

*Acceptance Groups for Survivors* are designed to be conducted in a series of 24 sessions, usually once or twice per week, each one hour in duration. The program is applicable to persons with disabilities from traumatic brain injury, other forms of traumatic injuries causing loss of function, or to persons with disabilities caused by diseases affecting the brain and central nervous system, such as Parkinson's disease, multiple sclerosis, and postpolio syndrome. Persons recovering from substance abuse or addictions of any kind also are "survivors" who benefit from Acceptance Groups.

Based on the life experience of brain-injury survivor Nancy Bauser, MSW, ACSW, this structured group program is designed to help survivors accept themselves the way they are, to learn to be honest with themselves and to "be comfortable in their own skin." Only such acceptance allows survivors to realistically assess where they are, where to begin their recovery and face the challenge of becoming stronger.

"Survivors need to figure out what currently limits them. They need to determine what they can't do and what they can. When the goal is to take their place in the mainstream, often moving in a straight line into the future is no longer possible," Ms. Bauser says.

Those who might make use of Acceptance Groups include rehabilitation specialists, counselors, social workers, neuro-psychologists, and psychologists working in inpatient or outpatient rehabilitation settings or independent living centers.

# Objectives of *Acceptance Groups for Survivors*

- Grasp the concept of acceptance as a process of recognizing problems, admitting deficits, and finally *accepting* the reality of the present moment — the process of acceptance is repeated throughout life in all difficult situations.

- Become invested in recovery by understanding that each individual defines his or her own recovery.

- Build an understanding of the need for "healthy interdependence," the need to support as well as be supported, and the need to be involved in activities each individual sees as worthwhile.

- Understand that personal worth is not determined by ability to function.

- Explore feelings accompanying disability.

- Deal with loss by learning how to grieve and let go.

- Become more aware of personal strengths and weaknesses.

- Begin to build a solid framework of realistic goals.

- Learn problem solving skills.

*Facilitators need to be aware that participants enter the groups with different levels of understanding, come from different backgrounds, and possess different intellectual abilities. Because of individual differences as well as diagnoses, each participant will progress at his or her own pace. Acceptance doesn't eliminate sadness. It simply helps people move through difficult circumstances.*

# A Message from the Author

ACCEPTANCE! What a misunderstood word that is. When I started leading groups to help survivors of brain injury learn to accept, value — and love — their new post-injury selves, I had no idea that what I was doing was so radical. It made so much sense to me. After many years of being a brain injury survivor and continuously struggling to create a new life for myself, shouldn't I help others who were seeking to do that same thing?

Those years taught me the key to recovery is acceptance. I learned that clearing each hurdle I faced took a three-step approach. First, I had to *recognize* I had a problem, recognize that a hurdle existed. By that I mean I had to notice a problem and think, "Yes, this may be a problem, but I'm not ready to deal with it now." Next, I had to *admit* to myself that I could no longer deny the problem — this obstacle was not going to magically disappear. Admitting a problem actually existed was a big step because it meant I had moved past denial and toward the final step, which would allow me to do something about the difficulty I was facing.

That third step, of course, is acceptance. I had to *accept* where I was, so I would allow myself to take the small, achievable steps that would improve some aspect of my behavior. Let me tell you a little more about my pre-injury self. In 1971, I was an active, liberal, rebellious college student at the University of Michigan in Ann Arbor. Very social, I was well organized, intelligent and goal-oriented. I was fiercely independent with just the right touch of passive-aggressive resistance to authority figures. "The times they were a-changing," and I was changing with them. I remember laughing a lot, handling stress without much anxiety and managing multiple demands with ease.

In the fall of that year, a head-on collision shattered my world. I became a patient. I had it all: CPR, full life support, coma, multiple fractures and a severe brain injury. I made my return to mainstream life slowly, with lots of setbacks along the way. At that time, there were no brain injury specialists, not that any medical professional of today would have made a fundamental difference — I had to find out on my own what people with disabilities all must eventually realize. My recovery depends most upon my own input. Doctors and therapists can only assist.

My recovery required persistence through devastating defeats. After finishing college, I lived in my parents' basement until I decided what I wanted to do next. I got my master's degree in social work, because graduate study came easily. I was fine as long as I could concentrate on one thing at a time. Holding a job was difficult. I had three different jobs as a social worker and was fired from each one. I then worked at a number of lesser jobs, left the state of Michigan in search of a new life, and returned home when I was unable to find what I had hoped for. At that time, I contacted Michigan Rehabilitation Services. I was a client of that agency at various times during the next six years. The agency finally placed me in a sheltered workshop where I worked for more than two years until I had a seizure — yet another setback I had to overcome.

Along the way, I had to accept my new self a little at a time. Immediately after the accident, my denial of disability dominated my life. Repeated failure eroded this denial. Improvement was not possible until I fully experienced what I had lost. When I was done grieving for lost abilities, I became ready to accept the losses and begin working on my recovery. My experiences through the years have taught me that I must continuously learn new information and acquire new skills. Though it takes me longer than others, I absolutely refuse to give up, no matter how long it takes to reach my goals.

I grieve differently today. Sometimes, I grieve for lost opportunities like the chance to have taken my place in workforce. I'm sad that I've lost the ability to concentrate or read for long periods of time and to organize detailed projects. Because of residual limitations, I realize there are activities I'm not able to do like the "old Nancy" would have done them, and that makes me sad. But, I don't grieve as long or as deeply as I used to. I accept the sadness and go on. As I get better and attempt new behaviors, I become more aware of losses that I previously did not recognize. So I now grieve more for lost potential.

In the end, I have come to realize that my recovery, just like my life, is dependent on what I make of it. To regain control over my life and my future, I first had to believe that I was a new person. Though similar to my pre-injury self, I was very different in some important ways. I had severe limitations that required my setting goals founded in my new reality.

Since 1986, my story has taken a happier turn. I met and later married my best friend. I have been able to capture some of the lessons I've learned and put them into this series called *Acceptance Groups for Survivors.* I now pay better attention to my limitations and am doing work that I both enjoy and am able to do well. That work is presenting my Acceptance Groups to survivors of injury/disability/illness caused by any life-changing event, physical or mental.

# Guidelines for Facilitators

Acceptance Groups are designed to be constructive, "sharing" sessions, not psychotherapeutic groups. Anyone who chooses to attend a session is welcomed and all participants are encouraged to speak at some point. Those who facilitate *Acceptance Groups for Survivors* should adhere to these rules:

- Allow new participants to join groups at any time. It is not necessary to begin with Week 1 and progress sequentially through the 24 groups.

- Stay positive. Groups are not meant to be sad gatherings of victims, but tools to help survivors discover ways they can live and prosper with whatever has happened to them. Lead complainers to look at situations from different, more positive perspectives.

- Avoid direct confrontations. Groups are *not* sessions meant for merely venting distressing emotions or displaying antisocial behaviors. Rather they are teaching opportunities to help people discover how they can live as independently as possible and attain goals within their personal limitations. Empathize with participants, but always attempt to lead them toward a positive outlook.

- Encourage the support and sharing of the full range of experiences of group members, not just those relating to resolving negative behaviors and feelings, but those moments in recovery that are positive, enriching and triumphant.

- Since people learn through repetition, begin every group with the same positive statements. **Begin every session** by asking one of the survivors/participants to read:

    **"Recovery does not mean that you will wake up one day and you're fine. It does not mean your memory becomes intact. It does not mean you don't get confused, and it certainly does not mean you regain the life you had prior to the injury/disability/ illness."**\*

    **Recovery to a person with an injury/ disability/illness is making progress. Making progress is ACCEPTING your**

**deficits, learning success "strategies to help you with those deficits, and learning to love and value yourself."**\*

---

\**Note:* (Quotations from *Gentle Touches* by Carol Taylor, February 1991)

Then, ask another survivor to read these rules:

# Rules for Group Behavior

1. We talk from our own experience.

2. We respect other's right to feel the way they feel.

3. What is said in Acceptance Group is confidential.

4. We treat others the way we wish to be treated.

5. There is no right or wrong way to feel.

- End every group on a positive note, as well. Participants, at first, may object, argue, express disapproval, but facilitators should **end every session** by asking **all** participants to make a positive statement about themselves or name one positive change they have made that is a result of their injury/disability/illness.

# Part I — Dealing with Me

The first six sessions in the structured group program *Acceptance Groups for Survivors* are designed to help participants understand the process of acceptance. These group sessions help participants address the issues of denial and avoidance and learn to assess their deficits and talk about them. Facilitators acknowledge participants' feelings, thus validating those feelings and helping to build self-esteem.

It is suggested that facilitators lead an interactive discussion of the questions listed, keeping in mind the methods discussed under "Guidelines for Facilitators" (page xxiii).

During Part I, facilitators should lead participants toward an understanding of the following

*Nancy Bauser M.S.W., A.C.S.W.*

concepts. These are the **key issues** that help survivors to regain and reclaim health.

*Recovery* — Survivors are the ones who need to define their own recoveries. Each person's definition of recovery will evolve as each individual builds upon his or her own successes. It is through this process that people change and grow.

*Acceptance* — Acceptance is coming to terms emotionally and intellectually with reality. It's a term that means different things at different times. It includes feeling satisfied by making a "best effort," regardless of the outcome. When one accepts, one is content and stops struggling to win battles that can not or need not be won.

*Expectations* — What is unrealistic today can only become possible after goals are set, worked for and achieved. It often is failing to meet one's expectations that causes pain, more than failing to achieve a particular goal.

***Independence*** — Complete independence is an ideal and impossible. Everyone needs interdependent relationships with family members, support persons, friends, co-workers and environments. Survivors need to become aware that others depend on them in order to see themselves as part of mutually supportive relationships. Understanding the need for **"healthy interdependence"** must be the goal here — learning that interdependence means standing alone *with some level of assistance.*

*Nancy Bauser M.S.W., A.C.S.W.*

# Notes

*Acceptance Groups for Survivors*

# Week 1: Meanings of Acceptance and Recovery

## Objectives:

- Establish a rapport among participants by talking to one another and discovering similarities in experiences and feelings.

- Verbalize individual definitions of recovery and acceptance.

- Build self-confidence by having opinions acknowledged as valid.

*Nancy Bauser M.S.W., A.C.S.W.*

## Questions for discussion:

1. What does it mean to recover?

2. How does recovery happen?

3. What does it mean to accept one's injury/disability/illness?

4. How does acceptance affect recovery?

5. What do you need to do to begin to accept and recover?

# Week 2: Expectations of Self

## Objectives:

- Consider the idea that group members need to change their expectations — begin to see that their injury/disability/illness has changed them and their pre-injury expectations will need to change accordingly.

- Learn expectations of perfection are not possible.

- Understand that they may no longer be able to "keep up with" their mainstream friends or associates. Learn that it is possible to accomplish things differently.

*Nancy Bauser M.S.W., A.C.S.W.*

- Understand that participants have strengths, in fact, have new strengths, and need to recognize and maximize these strengths.

## Questions for discussion:

1. What steps are you willing to take to recover?

2. What do you expect your life to be like now that you have become injured/disabled/ill?

3. Since your injury/disability/illness, what do you do and how do you feel when you seem to be left behind by your family, friends, or coworkers?

4. When is doing the best you can good enough?

5. How can you feel OK just the way you are?

*Nancy Bauser M.S.W., A.C.S.W.*

# Notes

# Week 3: Physical Limitations As a Result of Injury/Disability/Illness

## Objectives:

- Stop denying what has happened by verbalizing current physical and emotional limitations.

- Honestly express feelings of anger, rage and depression at what has happened.

*Nancy Bauser M.S.W., A.C.S.W.*

## Questions for discussion:

1. Do you know your physical limitations? What are they?

2. How do your limitations interfere with your daily functioning?

3. How do you feel about having "new" limitations?

4. How are you able to feel OK when your body will not do what you want it to do?

5. How do you reconcile yourself to your present state when mainstream America is so concerned with physical image?

## Week 4: Healthy Problem Solving

### Objectives:

- Realize group members are angry at the changes they must face because of their injury/disability/illness.

- Identify any maladaptive behaviors — isolating themselves, drinking, taking drugs, displacing anger, acting violently, binge eating, excessive shopping, or gambling — that are the result of attempts to cope with anger.

- Consider healthy ways of solving problems, such as taking on that which is difficult

*Nancy Bauser M.S.W., A.C.S.W.*

incrementally — prioritizing problems and working on small pieces individually.

## Questions for discussion:

1. How do you express your anger at your injury/disability/illness?

2. Which behaviors are ones that you can't stop once you start?

3. What relief do you get from engaging in those behaviors?

4. How can you solve problems in a healthy, beneficial way?

5. In a healthy way, how would you solve the problem of not getting something you wanted?

*Nancy Bauser M.S.W., A.C.S.W.*

## Notes

## Week 5: Living with an Injury/Disability/Illness

Objectives:

- Recognize behaviors that result from denial or attempts to get preferential treatment by assuming a "victim" status.

- Understand that participants' injury/disability/illness is a part of them, but does not define them. They still have abilities and strengths to carry on with life.

- Recovery is a continuum. What they are able to do at the current time is where they begin. Where they go, and how they progress, from this point is up to each individual.

*Nancy Bauser M.S.W., A.C.S.W.*

- Learn to ask for help when needed — total independence is unattainable; total dependence is undesirable. "Healthy" interdependence is the goal.

## Questions for discussion:

1. How do you tell others about your injury/disability/illness?

2. When do you define yourself by your difficulties? How could you explain yourself differently?

3. When do you get angry at yourself for having an injury/disability/illness? How do you express guilt or shame?

4. Were you accustomed to doing things by and for yourself before your injury/disability/illness? How has this changed?

*Nancy Bauser M.S.W., A.C.S.W.*

5. Who made the decisions that have directed your treatment and rehabilitation so far? How do you feel about that? What changes would you like to see made?

*Acceptance Groups for Survivors*

# Week 6: Dealing with Me — Review Weeks 1 to 5

## Objectives:

- Understand the process of acceptance.

- Move past denial so improvement can begin. Be able to verbalize current physical and emotional limitations.

- Become invested in recovering by defining paths to recovery.

- Understand the concept of healthy interdependence.

*Nancy Bauser M.S.W., A.C.S.W.*

## Questions for discussion:

1. What are steps you will take to recover from your losses?

2. What will you do when you are unable to live up to your own expectations of yourself?

3. Can you identify two new limitations and explain how you plan on living with them?

4. What do you need to know in order to solve a problem?

5. How would you describe yourself to someone you just met?

*Acceptance Groups for Survivors*

# Part II — Dealing With Others

These six sessions in the structured group program *Acceptance Groups for Survivors* are designed to help survivors develop social interaction skills, including understanding what a support system is, what it means to be a friend, and how and when to ask for help. Survivors also re-evaluate their expectations about work and build self-esteem by better understanding self-worth. Facilitators lead participants toward these objectives through interactive discussion of the questions listed. As in Part I, facilitators should follow the "Guidelines for Facilitators" (page xxiii).

The following concepts are the **key issues** participants confront during Part II in order to begin regaining and reclaiming health.

***Work/Volunteer Work*** — Being involved in activities (work) survivors see as worthwhile is crucial to their feeling any level of satisfaction. Sensing that they are a valuable part of something larger than themselves — whether or not they are receiving compensation — is why working is so important.

***Support System*** — Whether family, friends or the acceptance group itself, support systems are there to offer assistance. Recognizing support systems and how to work positively within them, survivors learn not to lose sight of their role in providing support as well as receiving support.

***Worth*** — Personal value or worth is best never equated to the amount of money made. Rather, worth involves all that survivors are and all that they do. By considering people who are most important to them, participants realize worth has little to do with money.

***Friendship*** — One of the rules of the group, read at the start of each session, is: "We treat others the way we wish to be treated." This rule is a defining quality of friendship. Realizing that friends give as well as take, support as well as receive support, survivors assess the quality of their friendships and appraise what they contribute to friendships they value. Finally, it's best when survivors understand that no matter what their life circumstances are, it is the nature of friendships to evolve and change with time.

*Nancy Bauser M.S.W., A.C.S.W.*

# Notes

## Week 7: Getting Back to Work

Objectives:

- Address the issues of denial and avoidance in relation to expectations about work. Understand the need to re-evaluate job goals.

- Consider volunteer work as a worthwhile means to re-learn or practice work habits and interactions with supervisors and co-workers.

- Build self-esteem by having feelings validated by the group and the facilitator.

*Nancy Bauser M.S.W., A.C.S.W.*

## Questions for Discussion:

1. Since your injury/disability/illness, what do you think you can do in the workplace?

2. How much money do you think you are presently worth to an employer? What leads you to that belief?

3. How long do you think you could work without a break?

4. Do you need to re-evaluate your job expectations?

5. How do you feel about volunteer work?

## Week 8:  Support Systems

Objectives:

- Explain what a support system is. Name people, groups and organizations that serve as support systems.

- Identify individual support systems. Learn that it's OK to ask for help when needed.

- Build participants self-esteem by discussing how feelings of worth are acquired, the reality of rejection and how to deal with both these realities.

*Nancy Bauser M.S.W., A.C.S.W.*

## Questions for discussion:

1. What is a support system and how do you begin to build one?

2. Who is in your support system?

3. How do you feel about needing support as an adult?

4. When do you allow yourself to ask for assistance?

5. How can a support system help with having an injury/disability/illness?

*Acceptance Groups for Survivors*

# Week 9: Asking for Assistance

## Objectives:

- Overcome the fear of not conforming or being different.

- Learn that being who they are is valuable — even if they are different from those in the mainstream. Being different does not mean not being good enough.

- Discuss difficulties asking for help. Realize asking for assistance when needed is appropriate.

- Define "survivor" as a strong individual. Survivors have worth because they face adversity and overcome problems.

## Questions for discussion:

1. How do you think others are influenced by the visibility of the residuals of your injury/disability/illness?

2. What are your feelings about your own worthiness?

3. What does the word "survivor" mean to you?

4. How and when do you ask for help?

5. How do you feel about needing assistance with daily routines?

*Nancy Bauser M.S.W., A.C.S.W.*

# Notes

## Week 10: Relating to Others

Objectives:

- Understand the concept of social isolation and break through participants isolation.

- Discuss friendships, how they naturally evolve and change, how friends give as well as take.

- Discuss common courtesy skills needed to interact with people and be a good friend. Use "Rules of Group Behavior" as examples, especially respecting others' feelings and treating other participants as they, themselves, want to be treated.

*Nancy Bauser M.S.W., A.C.S.W.*

- Realize the people in their acceptance group are a support system — the group is a safe place to practice social interaction skills.

## Questions for discussion:

1. Since your injury/disability/illness, how have your friendships changed?

2. When you feel lonely, what do you do?

3. Before you came to this group, how well did the phrase "social isolation" describe your situation and how has that changed?

4. How can you be a good companion?

5. How can a new friendship be maintained — or — How do you keep the friendships you have?

*Nancy Bauser M.S.W., A.C.S.W.*

# Notes

# Week 11: Requiring Assistance

## Objectives:

- Define the following:

  Independent — I care for myself.

  Dependent — I need you to take care of me.

  Interdependent — By combining our efforts, we can better take care of each other.

- Discuss merging of independence and dependence into interdependence.

- Realize that trying to recover is making progress. Realize that by attending this group, they are making progress.

*Nancy Bauser M.S.W., A.C.S.W.*

- Be realistic about how the future will not be the same as the past. Recognize changes they are making as survivors.

## Questions for discussion:

1. After your injury/disability/illness, how were you dependent on others?

2. How have you become more independent in your daily routines?

3. Which of your day-to-day tasks require some assistance?

4. How would you define "interdependence"? How are you interdependent with your environment?

5. How has your injury/disability/illness changed your plans or goals for your future?

*Nancy Bauser M.S.W., A.C.S.W.*

# Notes

## Week 12: Dealing With Others — Review Weeks 7 to 11

## Objectives:

- Re-evaluate expectations about work; consider volunteer work as a worthwhile means to re-learn work skills or practice work habits.

- Understand the concept of support systems.

- Build survivor self-esteem through the understanding of self-worth.

- Learn how and when to ask for help and understand the meaning of interdependence.

*Nancy Bauser M.S.W., A.C.S.W.*

- Learn what it means to be a good friend. Practice social interaction skills.

- Understand the concept of social isolation and break through survivor isolation.

## Questions for discussion:

1. What activities allow you to structure your time?

2. How does having a support system help you live with your injury/disability/illness?

3. What does "requiring assistance" say about you?

4. How will you remedy the situation of being alone when you don't want to be?

5. How are you interdependent with your environment?

*Note: Review questions are meant to be answered briefly.*

*Nancy Bauser M.S.W., A.C.S.W.*

# Notes

# Part III — Dealing with Feelings

These six sessions in the structured group program *Acceptance Groups for Survivors* are designed to help survivors understand the feelings they are experiencing as a result of their injury/disability/illness. Participants discuss loss, learn cognitively how powerful their feelings of loss can be and how they often act out these feelings through destructive behaviors. Survivors are encouraged to assess their capabilities realistically to learn how to compensate for their losses and to assist themselves in efforts to re-integrate into the mainstream. Facilitators lead participants toward these objectives through interactive discussion of the questions listed. As in Parts I and II, facilitators should follow the "Guidelines for Facilitators" (page xxiii). The following concepts are **key issues** participants confront during Part III.

*Change* — Change is never comfortable. Most people resist change because the tendency is strong to want life's circumstances to remain constant and thus familiar. The reality is, however, that the only constant in life is change. When life's circumstances shift, welcoming change as an opportunity to learn and grow is a positive means of dealing with the inevitability of change.

*Control* — Participants learn that life's circumstances are the result of decisions — some made by themselves, some by others. By tackling one problem at a time, survivors can begin to gain some control over their lives and resolve some of the complications caused by their injury/disability/illness.

*Loss* — People living with injuries/disabilities/illnesses are constantly reminded of their losses when seeing those around them who appear able-bodied. Participants learn that the visibility of loss has nothing to do with its severity. Survivors also learn to mourn their losses by going through the stages of grieving. Finally, participants realize that those around them (family, friends, co-workers) may need to grieve for the loss of what had been a comfortable status quo for them.

*Letting Go* — Letting go happens at the end of the grieving process. It involves the releasing of pain, anger and old ideas of how life was going to progress. Once survivors let go of old beliefs and negative feelings, they learn to fill the void those feelings have left with plans based in their new reality. In order to build feelings of self-worth,

*Nancy Bauser M.S.W., A.C.S.W.*

participants need to believe that they can grab onto a new reality when they let go of the old.

## Week 13: Feelings about Being Injured/Disabled/Ill

Objectives:

- Recognize that injury/disability/illness has changed their life circumstances.

- Promote well being by realistically assessing current capabilities as their baseline for improvement.

- Assess the importance of the reactions of others and how these reactions affect their perceptions of themselves.

- Think positively.

*Nancy Bauser M.S.W., A.C.S.W.*

## Questions for discussion:

1. How has your injury/disability/illness changed your life?

2. How are you similar to your pre-injury/disability/illness self? What has changed?

3. In what ways do you deny, discount or minimize your abilities?

4. What effect has your injury/disability/illness had on those close to you?

5. Name something you like about yourself today.

## Week 14: Feeling OK Today

**Objectives:**

- Realize that by working within their current limitations they achieve some level of control.

- Improve self-worth.

- Build group unity by identifying with others in the group.

- Discover new personal boundaries.

*Nancy Bauser M.S.W., A.C.S.W.*

## Questions for discussion:

1. Over which activities in your life do you have control?

2. How can you feel OK when you need to ask for help to do activities that you were used to doing by yourself before your injury/disability/illness?

3. In what situations do you sometimes feel sorry for yourself?

4. How can you feel "good enough" when you need support?

5. What do you need to do in order to feel OK just the way you are?

*Acceptance Groups for Survivors*

# Week 15: Feelings About Self

## Objectives:

- Realistically assess abilities and limitations.

- Recognize behaviors used to deny injury/disability/illness.

- Empower participants to re-integrate into the mainstream by using the group as a "safe" place to rehearse behaviors.

*Nancy Bauser M.S.W., A.C.S.W.*

## Questions for Discussion:

1. Think about your strengths and weaknesses since your injury/disability/illness? Name at least one of each.

2. When do you feel you are not as valuable, worthy, or capable as others?

3. What behaviors help you to deny your injury/disability/illness?

4. What do you do when you feel abandoned by others? How can you begin to reach out?

5. How do your feelings about yourself affect your ability to interact with those in the mainstream?

## Week 16: Loss and Acceptance

Objectives:

- Realize others have losses and that loss is a universal human experience.

- Understand how intense feelings of loss can be — understand cognitively what loss is and actually feel their own losses.

- Discuss suicide and death not only to discourage suicide attempts, but also to become aware that these thoughts are not uncommon when learning to cope with grief and loss.

*Nancy Bauser M.S.W., A.C.S.W.*

- Introduce the concept that accepting their circumstances is OK.

## Questions for discussions:

1. What does the word "loss" mean to you?

2. How has your injury/disability/illness altered your abilities? How do you start compensating for your differences in a healthy way?

3. How does the label "damaged goods" feel to you? Why does it feel that way?

4. Would death be better than living with your residual limitations?

5. How do you accept what your life has become since your injury/disability/illness?

*Nancy Bauser M.S.W., A.C.S.W.*

# Notes

*Acceptance Groups for Survivors*

# Week 17: Expressing Uncomfortable Feelings

## Objectives:

- Understand that blaming themselves, feeling guilty or ashamed is not justified or necessary.

- Recognize that group members act out their feelings of loss and shame in various ways and that destructive behaviors are often tied to feelings of loss.

- Consider how participants might make their situations more acceptable to themselves.

*Nancy Bauser M.S.W., A.C.S.W.*

## Questions for discussion:

1. Do you sometimes feel guilty about having had (or even caused) the accident that left you injured/disabled or about having contracted your illness?

2. When you feel sorrow and despair, what do you do?

3. How do you express your anger at your limitations?

4. How do you "act out" your feelings? Do you engage in behaviors that you can't stop once you start? Are you addicted to substances? Are you depressed? Do you get involved in hurtful relationships?

5. What can you do today to make your situation more acceptable to you?

*Nancy Bauser M.S.W., A.C.S.W.*

# Notes

## Week 18: Dealing With Feelings – Review Weeks 13 to 17

## Objectives:

- Recognize that injury/disability/illness has thoroughly changed their life circumstances.

- Assess the importance of the reactions of others and how these reactions affect how they feel about themselves.

- Understand how powerful their feelings of loss can be and how they act out their feelings through destructive behaviors.

- Promote well being and self-worth through positive thinking about their current abilities and how they can compensate for their losses.

*Nancy Bauser M.S.W., A.C.S.W.*

## Questions for discussion:

1. What has changed about you since your injury/disability/illness? How do you feel about your differences?

2. When you feel that your injury/disability/illness interferes with your ability to participate in life, what do you tell yourself and others?

3. When you feel angry, depressed or without energy, what do you do?

4. In what activities do you participate that allow you to feel OK just as you are?

5. Can you name three behaviors you engage in that assist you in compensating for your losses?

*Nancy Bauser M.S.W., A.C.S.W.*

# Notes

# Part IV — Putting It Together

The final six sessions in the structured group program *Acceptance Groups for Survivors* are designed to reinforce the key concepts introduced in Parts I through III. If survivors have participated in these first 18 sessions, they will have discovered attitudes and feelings they hold about themselves and others. They will now be more aware of their strengths and weaknesses and be better able to choose behaviors in which to participate as they begin to re-integrate into the mainstream. Specifically, these sessions are designed to help participants define:

***Themselves*** — Participants will see the need to take a closer look at themselves and redefine themselves based on all they have learned. The new definition will be sharper because it will be *based on facts* they have acknowledged, admitted and have begun to accept about their post injury/disability/illness selves.

***Their Goals*** — With an accurate picture of who they are, participants can begin to build a solid framework of realistic goals. Survivors need to understand that their setting goals has value — not only for themselves, but survivors' goal setting also has value for others in their lives.

***Their Plans and Methods*** — Armed with a clearer understanding of their new selves and a framework of realistic, achievable goals, survivors can begin constructing the stairway that will reach their goals. The steps in the stairway will consist of people who can assist them, friendly environments and familiar tools they can use.

## Week 19: Feeling Good About Yourself

### Objectives:

- Continue the ongoing process of acceptance by acknowledging, admitting, and then accepting their injury/disability/illness.

- Realize that dwelling on anger, guilt or shame, and acting out negative emotions will not help participants re-integrate into the mainstream.

- Be aware of what specific thoughts and activities help them cope best with their losses and feel good about themselves.

*Nancy Bauser M.S.W., A.C.S.W.*

## Questions for discussion:

1. What can you do to feel better about yourself today?

2. What has your injury/disability/illness cost you? What have you lost? Now, what are you willing to do about those losses?

3. In what activities do you participate that allow you to feel good about yourself now?

4. How can you begin to recover from your losses?

5. How do you learn to like yourself?

# Week 20: Possibilities After Injury/Disability/Illness

Objectives:

- Realistically assess limitations and abilities.

- Accept need for support.

- Identify feelings about life after injury/disability/illness.

*Nancy Bauser M.S.W., A.C.S.W.*

## Questions for Discussion:

1. Immediately after your injury or the onset of your disability or illness, was there a time when you were physically and/or mentally helpless? How has that changed?

2. In what areas do you still require support? How can that be OK?

3. What are your feelings about what your life will be like since your injury/disability/illness?

4. How does your injury/disability/illness actually affect what you do today?

5. How does your injury/disability/illness affect how you feel about yourself today?

## Week 21: Disability and the Workplace

Objectives:

- Verbalize strengths as they would for an employer; sell themselves to each other.

- Formulate answers to potential employers' and co-workers' questions about visible needs; rehearse answers in the group.

- Learn how to ask for and accept help, when needed. Understand the concept of inter-dependence.

*Nancy Bauser M.S.W., A.C.S.W.*

## Questions for discussion:

1. How do you feel about a potential employer knowing you have an injury/disability/illness?

2. How do you address or explain your strengths and deficits to that employer?

3. How do you feel about needing support on the job?

4. What will you tell your future co-workers about your visible needs?

5. How can you feel OK when you need help on the job?

*Acceptance Groups for Survivors*

# Week 22: Setting Limits

## Objectives:

- Recognize when deficits overshadow abilities; learn where to draw boundaries.

- Communicate honestly about deficits; learn not to be deceptive with themselves or others.

- Improve self-esteem; learn to like themselves despite limitations.

*Nancy Bauser M.S.W., A.C.S.W.*

## Questions for discussion:

1. What does it mean to set a limit for yourself?

2. Why establish limits?

3. What do you need to know to establish limits?

4. How do you make others aware of your special needs?

5. How can you feel OK when you have limitations?

# Week 23: Accepting Yourself Just the Way You Are

## Objectives:

- Understand the importance of self-worth and what makes them value themselves.

- Learn that life changes continuously at every age; change is difficult no matter what the circumstances.

- Recognize that reactions to life changes often are feeling responses that have little basis in reality and can be destructive.

- Learn recovery is making progress; it's an ongoing process.

*Nancy Bauser M.S.W., A.C.S.W.*

## Questions for Discussion:

1. How do you think your self-worth has been affected by your injury/disability/illness?

2. How does it feel to be injured/become disabled or ill at your age? What difference does age make in learning to accept and live with an injury/disability/illness?

3. How well do you risk change? Explain.

4. "It's not what happens to us, but our response to what happens to us that hurts us."* How does this statement apply to you?

---

*Stephen R. Covey, <u>The 7 Habits of Highly Effective People</u>, p.73

5. Does accepting yourself today mean that you will stop trying to regain lost abilities?

*Nancy Bauser M.S.W., A.C.S.W.*

# Notes

*Acceptance Groups for Survivors*

# Week 24: Putting It Together Review Weeks 19 to 23

## Objectives:

- Recognize personal progress; understand that positive change is possible.

- Verbalize how to ask for help, when needed.

- Realistically assess limits; know how to verbalize deficits.

- Accept themselves as they are; understand recovery is making progress.

*Nancy Bauser M.S.W., A.C.S.W.*

## Questions for Discussion:

1. In what activities do you participate now that allow you to feel good about yourself?

2. Name behaviors that were not possible for you after your injury/disability/illness that are possible today?

3. What do you say to yourself when you need help on the job? at home? with friends?

4. What are two of your personal limits?

5. How will accepting yourself today help your recovery?

*Acceptance Groups for Survivors*

# Notes

*Nancy Bauser M.S.W., A.C.S.W.*

# Notes

## Notes

*Nancy Bauser M.S.W., A.C.S.W.*

# Notes

# About the Author

Nancy Bauser, MSW, ACSW, is a survivor of a traumatic brain injury, which she sustained in an automobile accident in 1971. Following her injury, she had to relearn to walk, talk, and function independently. She went on nine months later to complete her undergraduate degree, and, subsequently, a graduate degree in social work. Since her accident, Ms. Bauser has lived for more than 30 years experiencing the triumphs and defeats that accompany living with a traumatic brain injury.

Ms. Bauser developed *Acceptance Groups for Survivors* out of her own life experience. This structured group program for survivors of brain injuries, disabling mental or physical diseases, and/or addictions is based on the concept of acceptance of one's life circumstances. It employs

*Nancy Bauser M.S.W., A.C.S.W.*

interactive discussion of a series of themes and questions common to survivors coping with disabilities. Ms. Bauser's work now includes peer counseling and conducting Acceptance Groups with survivors of brain injury and various psychological and traumatic disorders at outpatient treatment facilities in southeastern Michigan.

Printed in the United States
4113